Delia Luisa Sánchez Pacheco
Carlos Manuel González Brizuela
Alina Márquez Chacón

Allergen-specific sublingual immunotherapy

Delia Luisa Sánchez Pacheco
Carlos Manuel González Brizuela
Alina Márquez Chacón

Allergen-specific sublingual immunotherapy

Application on the basis of mites in bronchial asthma

ScienciaScripts

Imprint
Any brand names and product names mentioned in this book are subject to trademark, brand or patent protection and are trademarks or registered trademarks of their respective holders. The use of brand names, product names, common names, trade names, product descriptions etc. even without a particular marking in this work is in no way to be construed to mean that such names may be regarded as unrestricted in respect of trademark and brand protection legislation and could thus be used by anyone.

Cover image: www.ingimage.com

This book is a translation from the original published under ISBN 978-613-9-43863-1.

Publisher:
Sciencia Scripts
is a trademark of
Dodo Books Indian Ocean Ltd. and OmniScriptum S.R.L publishing group

120 High Road, East Finchley, London, N2 9ED, United Kingdom
Str. Armeneasca 28/1, office 1, Chisinau MD-2012, Republic of Moldova, Europe
Printed at: see last page
ISBN: 978-620-8-22662-6

SUMMARY

The book is an epidemiological, observational, analytical case-control study to identify variations in the effectiveness of allergen-specific sublingual immunotherapy with mites in persistent asthmatic patients who attended the Allergology Department of the Hospital Provincial Clínico "Saturnino Lora" in the province of Santiago de Cuba, in the period from January 2022 to 2024. The universe is made up of all patients who attended the outpatient consultation of the Allergology Service and met the established inclusion and exclusion criteria. For the selection of the sample, simple random sampling was used, forming two groups: study and control, **with** *a total of 132 patients participating in the study. The study group used sublingual immunotherapy with mites as part of the treatment, 44 patients, and the control group only used pharmacological treatment, 88 patients. The data were processed using the SPSS statistical system version 11.5 for Windows, presented in tables and graphs, and summary measures were used. To identify the statistically significant association, the Chi-square test of homogeneity was used. It is concluded that sublingual immunotherapy produces variations that responded to a decrease in symptomatology, a reduction in visits to emergency medical services, less use of rescue and controller medication, a decrease in nasal eosinophilia; they also presented less absenteeism from work and only local adverse reactions were reported, which positively influenced the control and improvement of the quality of life of these patients.*

INDEX

INTRODUCTION

Immunotherapy consists of the administration of increasing doses of an allergenic extract linked to the allergic process with the aim of achieving clinical and immunological tolerance.[1-4] Although controversial and debated, it remains the only potential cure for some allergic diseases such as rhinoconjunctivitis, asthma and hymenoptera stings.[2, 3] Recommendations from professional bodies range from cautious acceptance (Weeke 1991) to outright rejection (Henry 1990).[5, 6]
The origins of immunotherapy go back to the first immunisation studies conducted by Pasteur and Edward Jenner in 1796 who extracted pus from the hand of a milkmaid who had contracted smallpox and inoculated an eight year old boy, who developed mild local symptoms, approximately a month and a half later was inoculated with the dreaded disease and did not suffer from it, thus demonstrating the protection offered by the vaccine; Other studies also led to the development of highly effective vaccines that have virtually eradicated a wide range of diseases, including smallpox, polio, yellow fever, diphtheria, tetanus and whooping cough.[7- 10]

Immunotherapy for the treatment of allergic diseases is based on the work of Noon and Freeman, who in 1911 attempted the immunisation of hay fever patients with grass (pollen toxin) by means of serial subcutaneous injections of grass pollen extract, calculated on a weight basis (Noon units), in their opinion the mechanism of action consisted in the production of an antitoxin against a pollen toxin, thus introducing seasonal immunotherapy.[6, 7]

Freeman in 1914 published the first trial of immunotherapy in 84 patients treated with grass pollen and reported acquired immunity at least one year after treatment was discontinued.[7, 8]

In 1921, Prausnitz and Kustner discovered a certain serum factor that transferred allergic wheal and inflammatory reactions from one individual to another.[9-12] Researchers such as Cooke and Coca followed, who in 1923 introduced the term atopy, and reported the presence of antibodies they called "reagins", they further demonstrated that patients treated with allergen injections subsequently developed blocking antibodies having the ability to inhibit the passive transfer reaction. This antibody was later shown to be an immunoglobulin G.[13-16]

The discovery in 1967 by Ishizaka and Johansson,[6] of the immunoglobulin IgE as reagin described above establishes its major role in inflammation in allergic diseases. The significance of specific IgE in diagnosis by skin tests and in vitro determinations and its neutralisation by immunotherapy. This research has made it possible to define allergy today as a hypersensitivity reaction initiated by immunological mechanisms and mediated by antibodies or cells.[7, 17-21]

Specific immunotherapy is one of the cornerstones of respiratory allergy treatment, alongside pharmacological treatment and allergen avoidance, and has long been a controversial treatment for asthma.[2, 6, 7] Since its introduction a century ago (1911),[6] has been administered subcutaneously, considered the conventional route of administration, but over the last two decades, the sublingual route has gradually been introduced into clinical practice, with the main aim of improving safety and convenience.[4-7]

The efficacy of sublingual immunotherapy has been demonstrated in numerous clinical trials and confirmed by several meta-analyses.[1, 3-8] Although some aspects still need to be clarified, it is considered a suitable therapeutic option and is widely used in Europe and other countries in different geographical latitudes.[4, 6, 8, 22-25]

Abramson et al. in 1995 published the first meta-analysis on the efficacy of allergen-specific immunotherapy in the treatment of asthma and in 1999 reported their latest meta-analysis on Immunotherapy, which included 62 papers published between 1954 and 1998, with irrefutable results on the subject.[5-11]

Skin tests were first described in 1873 by Blackley, and are the basis for specific immunotherapy, followed by Von Pirquet, Noon and Freeman, Cooke with scarification, scratching and more recently by Pepys himself in 1970 with the modified prick test technique.[4, 10, 26-30]

In our country the practice of Allergology began in the 1940s, practiced by about twenty doctors, not all of whom were allergists. The Cuban Society of Allergy was founded in 1949, and by 1960 the production of vaccines made from domestic dust began, and it was not until 1967 that Dr. Fernández de Castro proposed the use of bacterial vaccines with microorganisms from our environment.[8, 31-35]

On May 4, 1973 the first 6 specialists in allergology in our country graduated, and one of the thesis topics was "Sublingual hyposensitisation".[8, 33, 36, 37]

In 1992, the National Centre for Biopreparations (BIOCEN) was founded and since 2002 it has been producing allergenic extracts for puncture diagnosis, and since 2005 for therapeutic vaccines (immunotherapy), registered as VALERGEN® , the only industrial-scale manufacturer of this type of product in Cuba, and the first standardised allergenic products registered in Latin America.

In 2007 it began to be distributed in the national drug network and in 2008 it was officially included in the basic drug list.[37-40]

These are standardised products in biological units of the most common mite species in the tropical and subtropical environment, with a lyophilised presentation that guarantees absolute stability of the product in its composition and potency, including dermatophagoides pteronyssinus, dermatophagoides siboney and blomia tropicalis mites, which are widely used in our allergological services. [39,40]

Sublingual immunotherapy induces profound modifications in the immune response to allergens involving regulatory T cells, cytokines and effector cells.[29, 30] This complex mechanism of action results in a reduction of inflammatory phenomena in target organs, with a multi-organic, long-lasting, preventive, clinical and immunological tolerance-inducing action.[1-3, 12, 13, 17, 21]

It has been proposed that during sublingual immunotherapy Langerhans (dendritic) cells capture the allergen in the oral mucosa where they naturally express high and low affinity receptors for immunoglobulin E and produce IL-10 and TGF-β and thereby act on T-cell production, subsequently these cells mature and migrate to proximal lymph nodes. These local lymph nodes may favour the production of blocking IgG antibodies and the induction of suppressor lymphocytes.[11, 12, 21, 23-25]

The changes induced in the immune response give rise to special properties not shared by the drugs, such as the preventive effect and the long-term persistence of clinical benefits after discontinuation of immunotherapy, thus suggesting the modification of the natural course of the disease with regard to the protective effect against the development of new sensitisations.[2, 4, 8, 31-34]

The efficacy of oromucosal immunotherapy has been discussed for some years. In the last two years, several studies have been published supporting its usefulness in the treatment of rhinoconjunctivitis and bronchial asthma of allergic cause, both in children and adults. The allergenic extract is administered sublingually for one or two minutes and then swallowed, so that some of the extract is also absorbed through the stomach.[5-7, 31, 32]

The fact that sublingual immunotherapy requires the extract to be swallowed to be effective indicates that the immune system of the digestive system also plays a role.[31-33]

Allergens are administered for absorption through the surface of the oral mucosa, which is considered immunologically privileged as it is in constant contact with countless antigens from food, commensal flora and various pathogenic microorganisms that come into contact at this level, thereby inducing a form of special immunological tolerance, decreasing the local effector response.[20, 23-26, 34]

The target of immunotherapy must be controlling and specific:

- **Controlling (global):** Immunotherapy is part of the treatment of allergy as an aetiological factor, but must be complemented by adequate environmental control and appropriate preventive and symptomatic treatment.

- **Particular:** All environmental control measures and preventive and symptomatic treatments should be tailored to the needs of the individual patient at each stage of the process.[18, 29, 31-35]

Sublingual immunotherapy opens new avenues for improving asthma treatment and improving patients' quality of life, is being developed to increase safety and adherence to treatment, and is becoming increasingly potent, based on experimental data. It has been accepted by the World Health Organisation (WHO) and EAACI/ESPACI as a viable alternative.[11, 29, 30-35] It has been widely used in the last five years in different countries such as Italy, China, Japan, United Kingdom, Mexico, among others.[41-44]

Bronchial asthma has continuously occupied medical attention since antiquity (460-130 BC) and was referred to by Hippocrates, Galen and Aretaeus of Cappadocia. Celsus (30 B.C.E.) gave the name to the "moderate shortness of breath" experienced by soldiers during exercise.[8, 19]

There are an estimated 300 million people with the disease worldwide, and the health costs associated with asthma have been estimated at 11.5 million in direct costs and $4.6 million in indirect costs.[19, 35, 43]

The number of years lost, adjusted for disability, is estimated at around

15 million per year worldwide, one in 250 deaths are due to bronchial asthma, with considerable direct and indirect economic costs. With a projected increase in the world's urban population from 45 to 59 per cent by 2025, there will be more than 100 million additional asthmatics.[18, 19]

In 2008, a prevalence rate of 87.4 per 1 000 inhabitants was found in our country, with an estimated 980 210 asthmatic patients, which according to the number of inhabitants in the country, gives an asthma prevalence rate of 8.7 %.[35, 38]

Allergic conditions are the result of a complex interaction between genetic and environmental factors. Increasing experimental evidence indicates that continuous exposure, followed by sensitisation to house dust mites, is the primary cause of allergic asthma in many parts of the world.[37-41]

Their distribution in the human environment is influenced by numerous factors such as: geographical location, climate, lifestyles, building characteristics and the degree of modernisation and industrialisation, as a consequence their worldwide prevalence varies.[21, 22, 40-44]

The role of inhalant allergens (aeroallergens) in the exacerbation of respiratory allergies has been demonstrated, and within these the role of perennial allergens, with mites being the most interesting in this group; they are microscopic, 0.3 mm long, blind, photophobic arthropods, taxonomically related to spiders and ticks, which can be grouped into: domestic, storage and minor.[21, 22, 38, 40-44]

Numerous species have been isolated, but from an allergenic point of view, Dermatophagoides pteronyssinus and Dermatophagoides farinae, with their main allergens Der p and II and Der f I and II respectively, are of major importance.

Mites cohabit with humans in the domestic environment, mainly in dust accumulated in beds, mattresses, clothes, upholstered furniture and carpets. In our country the former predominates and in North America the latter, although they cross-react with each other. This is conditioned by the high relative humidity throughout the year, which also leads to the proliferation of storage mites. The two main factors that determine the growth and viability of mites are humidity and ambient temperature.[15, 21, 22]

Optimal conditions for mite growth are a temperature of 20-25 °C and a relative humidity of 75-85%, they are much less prevalent in dry and cold regions, in contrast to humid and temperate coastal areas, with our country as a tropical island being the ideal environment for their proliferation.[21, 22, 32, 34, 35-40, 44-48]

The association between hypersensitivity to environmental aeroallergens and asthma has been known for a long time. Nowadays, when airway inflammation is of particular interest in the definition of bronchial asthma, it has been shown that inhalation of aeroallergens, in sufficient quantity and time in sensitised individuals, is capable of inducing inflammation.[49-52]

Exposure to the allergen and the subsequent immuno-inflammatory response in the airways are phenomena that establish a clear cause-effect relationship between exposure and asthmatic disease.[53,54]

The variation in the amount of aeroallergens inhaled over time modifies the degree of inflammation and bronchial hyperresponsiveness and modulates the intensity of symptoms and can trigger asthma attacks. It is necessary to know the sensitisation or non-sensitisation of a given patient to the usual aeroallergens, as well as the allergenic pressure experienced by the subject over time.[10, 21, 22, 32, 34-38, 48-50] In daily practice, the efficacy of immunotherapy is generally demonstrated by a reduction in the symptoms of the disease that required specific treatment (asthma, rhinitis, rhinoconjunctivitis) and/or by a reduction in the need to use medication to combat the symptoms.[5, 6, 21, 24-26]

Allergen-specific sublingual immunotherapy in bronchial asthma has only recently been introduced and is a route of administration that simplifies treatment, as it can be carried out at home by the patient and can be administered by the patient himself. adverse effects are almost exclusively limited to the local area and severe anaphylactic reactions do not occur.[34, 40, 44, 47, 49]

Several studies support its efficacy, but there is a lack of studies demonstrating its action on the abnormal immune response of patients. The variation in serum levels of total and specific IgE and IgG4 after a period of treatment has been evaluated by several authors, but the results are contradictory and therefore not definitive.[49, 51-52]

In our environment, we are no strangers to the global behaviour of allergic diseases and especially bronchial asthma, which has a high prevalence in our country and in Santiago de Cuba; the growing number of patients suffering from it in all age groups with the need for increasingly frequent rescue treatments at high doses, the development of corticodependence and resistance, the considerable increase in triggering factors generally related to climatological and environmental changes, pollution and excessive urbanisation, motivate the relevance of this study. In the first half of this year, the allergy clinic of the "Saturnino Lora" Provincial Hospital, created in 1974, attended 4142 patients, 35% of whom suffer from bronchial asthma with different levels of severity. Of these, 8% receive conventional subcutaneous immunotherapy with VALERGEN, and no studies have been carried out to evaluate the efficacy of sublingual immunotherapy with mites in adult asthmatic patients.

This modality began to be used in the service in September 2010; an epistemological gap that generates the present research. With this background, from the holistic configurational model, we propose as a **Scientific Problem:** Deficiencies in the comprehensive management of adult asthmatic patients, which demonstrate the need to demonstrate the effectiveness of allergen-specific sublingual immunotherapy with mites in asthmatic patients classified as mild and moderate persistent from the clinical evolutionary point of view, as an affordable alternative that will contribute to a better management of asthmatic patients. better control of the disease and which will have a positive impact on the quality of life of these patients.

OBJECTIVE

To identify variations in the effectiveness of allergen-specific sublingual immunotherapy with mites in persistent asthmatic patients seen at the Allergology Clinic of the Saturnino Lora Provincial Hospital from January 2022 to 2024.

METHODOLOGICAL DESIGN OF THE RESEARCH

Bioethical considerations

All ethical considerations were taken into account when conducting this research, respecting the individuality of each patient at all times, maintaining total confidentiality regarding the results obtained in the surveys, starting with a detailed review of the individual clinical histories and, once the sampling had been carried out, the informed consent form (Annex I) was requested to participate in the research. It is based on the principle of achieving complete information for all patients with elements offered by the author of the work in an adequate and truthful manner, using clear language and understandable terminology to offer sufficient information in quantity and depth, all of which made it possible to understand the scope and consequences of participation in the research.It was taken into account that the individual would understand the information provided from his or her angle, according to his or her intelligence, reasoning ability, maturity and language, and at all times the principle of voluntariness prevailed, allowing patients to freely decide whether or not they wished to continue with the research. There was no coercion at any time when making decisions, in compliance with internationally endorsed ethical principles. The research was approved by the Ethics Committee for Scientific Research and the Scientific Council of the Saturnino Lora Provincial Hospital.

General characteristics of the research

An epidemiological, observational, analytical, case-control, public health research study was carried out to identify variations in the effectiveness of sublingual allergen-specific immunotherapy with mites in mild and moderate persistent asthma patients attending the Allergology Department of the Saturnino Lora Surgical Clinical Teaching Hospital in the Province of Santiago de Cuba, from January 2022 to 2024.

Methodical

The **universe** consisted of all patients who attended the outpatient clinic of the Allergology Service of the Hospital Provincial Saturnino Lora, in the period from January 2022 to 2024, with a diagnosis of mild and moderate persistent bronchial asthma, who met the following inclusion criteria:

Inclusion Criteria:

- Patients residing in the study area.

- Patients with a history of mild and moderate persistent bronchial asthma with regular follow-up and treatment in our Allergology Department.
- Patients of both sexes aged between 20 and 59 years.
- Patients with skin prick tests with Valergen DP, DS or BT 1/20 000 UB ≥ 3 mm (sensitisation to mites in our environment).

They are excluded from the study:

- Patients with decompensated chronic non-communicable diseases: neoplasms, collagenopathies, arterial hypertension, cardiopathies, nephropathies, psychiatric disorders, immunodeficiencies.
- Patients treated in the last two years with mite or dust mite allergen extracts.
- Patients who have discontinued immunotherapy for more than 30 days, with a history of previous severe systemic adverse reactions to skin tests or immunotherapy.
- Pregnant women.

- Patients with contraindications to the use of adrenaline, or who use beta-blockers as a regular and irreplaceable treatment.

For the selection of the sample, simple random sampling was used, forming 2 groups: study and control, with a total of 132 patients participating in the study, which corresponds to 77.6% of the universe.

The **study group** consisted of those patients with mild to moderate persistent asthma who were treated for 1 year with:
- Environmental Control Measures.

- Allergen-specific sublingual immunotherapy with VALERGEN allergen extracts.
- Rescue therapy in exacerbations: Short-acting B2 agonists (salbutamol) aerosolised or spray on demand.
- Inhaled steroids: Fluticasone spray: doses ranged from 250 to 500

micrograms daily.
Forty-four patients are included.

The **control group** consisted of those patients with mild to moderate persistent asthma who were treated for 1 year:
▪Environmental Control Measures.

▪Rescue therapy in exacerbations: Short-acting B2 agonists (salbutamol) aerosolised or spray on demand.
▪Inhaled steroids: Fluticasone spray: doses ranged from 250 to 500 micrograms daily. 88 patients were included.

Techniques and Procedures:

As a procedure for the collection of information, patients were interviewed face-to-face during the consultation, the allergological medical records were reviewed and/or drawn up, which constituted the primary source of information, and the data of interest for the study were entered in a primary data collection form created for this purpose (Annex II).An exhaustive interrogation and physical examination was included, as well as the indication of complementary examinations: complete blood count, global eosinophil count, erythrocyte sedimentation, faeces, glycaemia, lipidogram with cholesterol, triglycerides and hepatic profile, urea, creatinine, uric acid; from the immunological point of view, antibodies were quantified: IgA, IgM, IgG and total IgE, Serology and HIV, in addition, chest and sinus X-rays, cytological, bacteriological and BAAR sputum, cytology or nasal smear, respiratory functional test, nasopharyngeal exudate and electrocardiogram. Interconsultation with the specialities of Psychology, Otolaryngology, Cardiology and Internal Medicine was carried out. An interview was conducted with a guide of questions, most of which were taxative and included sociodemographic, clinical and other variables of interest to the study. Observation was used as the empirical method and analysis and synthesis as the theoretical method.The patients were scheduled for the next consultation in fifteen days, where they were fully evaluated with the results of the indicated complementary tests, and those who did not meet the established criteria were excluded from the study. The patients included in the study were given a Prick Test, with an explanation of the procedure, objectives and precautions to be taken into account before the test was performed.

They received regular bimonthly follow-up by the author of the research on pre-established days, with their individual clinical history, the model provided for the application of sublingual immunotherapy (Annex III) and the record card created to monitor symptoms and medication on a daily basis (Annex IV).

Patients in the study group were shown the technique of administering the immunotherapy, under the tongue, fasting, waiting 1 to 2 minutes and then swallowing, staying off food and water for the next 30 minutes, daily for the first 21 days during the build-up or induction phase, with bi-weekly maintenance from the fourth week onwards. The possible adverse reactions and the behaviour in case of adverse reactions, as well as the duration of the immunotherapy as a treatment for 3 to 5 years were warned about. At the sixth month, first and second year of treatment, clinical and humoral evaluation of the patients was carried out again, specifying the behaviour of the variables of interest for the study.

Definition of the variables under study

➢ **Socio-demographic variables:**

I.-Age: continuous quantitative variable, expressed in years, grouped into four class intervals of 10 years each:

▪ From 20 to 29 years old

▪ From 30 to 39 years old

▪ From 40 to 49 years old

▪ From 50 to 59 years old

The upper limit was 59 years because from this age onwards there are changes (involution) in the immune system that decrease its reactivity to skin tests and response to immunotherapy treatment, thus avoiding the inclusion of bias in the research.

II.- Sex: bimodal qualitative nominal or dichotomous variable. Biological sexes were considered, expressed as:

▪ Female

▪ Male

➢ **Variables related to the effectiveness of sublingual allergen-specific mite immunotherapy in persistent asthma patients. Nominal qualitative. They were classified into:**
I.**Clinical variables related to the modification of the natural course of the disease: These include:**
A. **Variables related to allergen sensitisation at baseline and one year after treatment, used only for the study group where sublingual mite immunotherapy was applied:**

Skin prick test or Prick Test:

Skin prick test on the right forearm, using allergen extracts for prick diagnosis at 20 000 BU/ml and two controls: positive (histamine hydrochloride solution at 1mg/1cc) and negative (diluent solution).

This diagnostic test is used to confirm or exclude the presence of allergen-specific IgE antibodies. It is one of the most widespread epicutaneous tests because of the advantages it offers: it is painless, low risk, several extracts can be tested simultaneously, immediate results and easy to perform.

Small amounts of the allergenic extract are introduced into the surface layer of the skin and upon diffusion into the surrounding tissue cause an IgE-mediated reaction in sensitised individuals, leading to the release of histamine and other mediators by epidermal mast cells, resulting in a characteristic wheal and erythema reaction at the site of application within 15-20 minutes.

The skin prick test was performed according to the procedures described below:
1. One drop of each allergen extract was applied to the right forearm.
2. The stainless steel lancet with a 1 mm tip was inserted through the droplet at a 30-45□ angle to the skin, then the lancet was removed and the excess droplet gently blotted with cotton wool.
3. Twenty minutes after the puncture, the test was read, the wheal produced at the puncture site was outlined with a pen.
4. The average diameter was measured with a millimetre ruler, resulting from the sum of the largest diameter of the wheal (maximum distance between the inner edges), and the orthogonal diameter (maximum distance between the edges, perpendicular to the largest diameter obtained at its midpoint) and divided by two. The area of erythema and

the presence of pseudopods were considered, which gave higher positivity to the tests.

5. A positive result was considered when the diameter of the wheal for the allergenic extract was greater than or equal to 3 mm, and negative when it was less than 3 mm.

List of products:

✓ Products under study:

1. Dermatophagoides pteronyssinus (VALERGEN-DP), Blomia tropicalis (VALERGEN-BT) and Dermatophagoides siboney (VALERGEN-DS) lyophilised and standardised in Biological Units (BU) (Potency: 20 000 BU/ml). The extract is presented in vials containing 100 000 BU and is made up in 5 ml of Diluent Solution, to obtain the concentration of 20 000 BU/ml.

✓ Control products:

1. Negative test control: restitution solution: phosphate buffer solution containing 0.4 % phenol and 0.03 % human serum albumin. It was also used as a solvent for the lyophilised extract.

2. Positive test control: Histamine hydrochloride solution with a concentration of 1mg/ml. Dropper bottle with 3 mL.

Product safety:

All products were stored refrigerated at 2-8°C temperature. The reconstituted allergen extracts were used for 6 months. The products were handled exclusively by the staff involved in the study (author, tutor, allergist-trained nurse, biologist and laboratory technician of the department).

A. Depending on the results of the skin prick test, patients were classified as follows:

▪ **Monosensitised:** Patient with sensitisation to one of the intradomiciliary mites tested: dermatophagoides pteronyssinus mite, dermatophagoides siboney, blomia tropicalis with a wheal area ≥ 3 mm, 20 minutes after the prick test, with no other sensitisation.

▪ **Bisensitised:** Patient with sensitisation to two of the intradomestic mites tested: dermatophagoides pteronyssinus mite, dermatophagoides siboney, blomia tropicalis: area of the wheal ≥ 3 mm, 20 minutes after the prick test, without other sensitisation.

- **Polysensitised:** Patient with sensitisation to more than two of the intradomestic mites tested: dermatophagoides pteronyssinus mite, dermatophagoides siboney, blomia tropicalis: area of the wheal ≥ 3 mm, 20 minutes after the prick test, without other sensitisation.

B. Variables related to the variation or appearance of new allergenic sensitisations. Nominal qualitative.

The initial diagnosis was taken into account, considering variation of the same when:

- **Negative reactivity:** Appearance of wheal or erythema < 3 mm, for all allergens tested in comparison with the control, no new sensitisation is recorded.
- **Decreased reactivity compared to the initial skin tests:** less wheal or erythema compared to the initial diagnosis, no negative reaction to all allergens tested and no new sensitisation.
- **Unchanging skin test reactivity:** Patients maintain the erythema or wheal obtained in the initial skin prick test performed, but no new sensitisation appears.
- **New reactivity:** Appearance of new sensitisations, which include not only other mites compared to the initial one, but also other aeroallergens such as anemophilic fungi.

C. Variables related to symptomatology according to severity: nominal qualitative.

Symptoms were considered to be the appearance during treatment of cough, fluid hyaline rhinorrhoea, nasolacrimal obstruction and/or pruritus, thick whitish expectoration, expiratory dyspnoea, chest tightness, wheezing or chest sounds, for which we used a symptom diary that was recorded on a record card created for this purpose (Annex V).

The frequency of symptom occurrence and the use of rescue medication were recorded per day, with a summary clause at the end of each day. month, that is assessed at the consultation at follow-up visit stratified by symptomatology as follows:

- Level 1: Daytime symptoms less than once a week and nocturnal symptoms no more than twice a month.

- Level 2: Daytime symptoms more than once a week but less than once a day, nocturnal symptoms occur more than twice a month.
- Level 3: Daily daytime symptoms, and nocturnal symptoms more than once a week.
- Level 4: Frequent daily and nocturnal daytime symptoms, almost daily with clinical picture of nocturnal asthma.

D. Variables related to the limitation of activities. Nominal qualitative:

Physical activity, from short walks to long distance running, was taken into account, assessing the need for premedication with short-acting bronchodilators such as salbutamol 30 minutes beforehand, or the use of inhaled steroids at least one week beforehand as a controller treatment.

They were reflected as follows:

- **No limitations:** Can perform any aerobic or non-aerobic physical exercise, symptom-free and does not use premedication with bronchodilators or inhaled anti-inflammatory drugs.
- **Mild limitation:** Perform short duration exercises from 30 minutes to one hour such as running, swimming, walking and aerobics, without the use of premedication.
- **Moderate limitation:** 5 to 10 block walks and short runs of 50 metres, long runs such as 800 metres slowly (2 laps of a running track) and prior medication (30 min before the start) with Beclomethasone and/or Salbutamol.
- **Severe limitation:** Unable to perform physical exercise because of lack of control of the disease, despite the use of anti-inflammatory premedication and/or bronchodilators.

E. Variables related to the number of visits to the emergency department in the year: Nominal qualitative.

All on-call attendances at the main emergency polyclinic or hospital for uncontrolled bronchial asthma (acute bronchial asthma attacks), or other complications derived from asthma, were considered, using the method indicated by the physician or the discharge form issued by the care centre in the case of admission, all grouped as follows:

- **Negative:** No emergency visits.

- **Slight positive:** Up to fourvisits aemergency department withou hospital admissions.

▪ **Medium positive:** Six ED attendances with at least 1 hospital admission that was not to the Intensive Care Unit.

▪ **Strong positive:** More from seven visits a emergency room with hospital admissions including admissions to the Intensive Care Unit.

F. Variablesrelated to work absenteeism due to bronchial asthma: Qualitative nominal:

▪ **Absent:** Patient who has never been absent from work or up to four absences per year due to bronchial asthma.

▪ **Present:** Patient with five and more annual absences due to bronchial asthma.

G. Variables related to lung function: Nominal qualitative: The results of forced spirometry were taken into account, which was indicated at the beginning of the study and was carried out at the Department of Respiratory Functional Testing at the "Dr. Juan Bruno Zayas" Clinical Surgical Teaching Hospital in Santiago de Cuba.

Forced spirometry is the manoeuvre that records the maximum volume of air that a subject can move from maximum inspiration to complete exhalation (i.e. until only the residual volume remains in the lungs). All expiratory manoeuvres were performed according to the protocol established by the referral service, interpreted as:

▪ Normal.

▪ Restrictive ventilatory disorder.

▪ Obstructive ventilatory disorder.

▪ Mixed ventilatory disorder

Also considered: Forced expiratory volume in the first second of expiration (FEV1): this is the volume of air expelled during the first second of forced expiration, in practice it is a measure of flow. It is considered normal if it is greater than 80% of its theoretical value.

FEV1/FVC ratio: This indicates the proportion of the FVC that is expelled during the first second of the forced expiratory manoeuvre. It is the most important parameter for assessing whether there is an obstruction, and under normal conditions it should be greater than 75%, although figures of up to 70% are accepted as non-pathological.

In our study we took into account for the interpretation of spirometry:

1. **Normal:** Improvement in lung function was confirmed in those patients who had an FEV1 and FEV1/FVC: ratio greater than 80% of the predicted value.
2. **Equal:** Patients who showed stability of lung function as they maintained FEV1 and FEV1/FVC ratio equal to the value found at the beginning of the investigation, i.e. no variability.
3. **Worsened:** Patients with impaired or decreased lung function with FEV1 variability and FEV1/FVC ratio less than 75%.

H. Variables related to the use of rescue medication. Qualitative Nominal:

Rescue medication is considered to be pharmacological groups with actions during exacerbations of bronchial asthma both in the early and late asthmatic response, to counteract effects such as: bronchoconstriction, oedema, inflammation, bronchial hyperreactivity. Among them are bronchodilators such as B2 agonists, in our environment salbutamol is used both in spray and aerosol, as well as aminophylline which is presented in 250 mg/ 10 cc ampoules for use in the treatment of bronchial asthma. intravenous. Anti-inflammatory drugs such as steroids used parenterally and/or orally, including hydrocortisone, prednisolone for intravenous or intramuscular use and prednisone 5 and 20 milligrams orally. These drugs were used in on-call corps, prescribed by medical staff. It was considered:

▪ **Non-use:** Patients who did not require rescue medication for exacerbations.

▪ **Use:** Patients who needed rescue medication regardless of dosage, frequency and intensity of the asthma attack.

I. Variables related to inhaled corticosteroid sparing (controller medication): Qualitative Nominal.

Controller drugs are those with topical anti-inflammatory action and low systemic potency, thus reducing mucosal inflammation and specific and non-specific bronchial hyperresponsiveness, protecting against early and late asthmatic response, improving lung function, and maintaining the disease without exacerbations or with reduced exacerbations.

Therefore, they should be administered daily, the main route of administration being inhalation, which reduces side effects, given the low percentage that is absorbed systemically (less than 1 %). Fluticasone spray was used as an inhaled steroid, with a minimum dose for adults of 250 to 500 micrograms per day, for a total of 2 to 4 puffs per day with a frequency of 1 to 4 times on average, and a maximum dose of 750 to 1000 micrograms per day, with 2 to 4 applications per dose administered every 4 hours, grouped into:

▪ **Section I:** Use of fluticasone spray doses of 750 to 1000 micrograms daily (maximum dose, 6 to 8 puff).

▪ **Section 2:** Use of beclomethasone spray doses of 375 to 500 micrograms per day, 3 to 4 puff.

▪ **Section 3:** Use of beclomethasone spray doses of 125 to 250 micrograms per day (minimum dose, 1 to 2 puff).

▪ **Section 4:** Non-use of inhaled steroids.

J. Variables related to Immunoglobulin E levels: Qualitative Nominal:

All those included in the study underwent determination of total serum immunoglobulin E (IgE), 5 mL of blood samples were taken and processed in the ENSUMA laboratory of the "Saturnino Lora" Provincial Clinical and Surgical Teaching Hospital. The UMELISA IgE programme was used: reagent for the quantitative determination of IgE in human serum developed by the national immunoassay centre.

Validation and interpretation of the results are performed automatically by the programme. Taking into account the different genetic and environmental factors that act on populations from different geographical locations and the variations that IgE levels can have in humans due to factors such as age, the presence of atopy and/or parasitic diseases, viral and fungal infections, international practice recommends that each laboratory establishes its own reference values.

Reference values: adults 150 IU/mL, with levels at or below normal and high above normal.

✓ **Adequate:** IgE levels below baseline, even if the value considered normal (150 IU/mL) was not obtained.

✓ **Inadequate:** IgE levels are high relative to baseline regardless of whether they were within the normal range.

K. Variables related to the local inflammatory response mediated by nasal eosinophils: Nominal qualitative:

Eosinophils are cells of the immune system that play an important role in bronchial asthma, which is why many authors have called the disease "eosinophilic desquamative bronchitis", they perpetuate the asthmatic response and its symptomatic manifestations. They are responsible for the late asthmatic response, which is why we consider it important to evaluate their behaviour according to nasal cytology results as a marker of inflammation at the beginning of the study and one year after immunotherapy:

They were assessed at baseline and at one year post-treatment and grouped as follows:

- **Reduction:** Number of eosinophils in nasal cytology normal or reduced by the percentage found at baseline.
- **Same:** Number of eosinophils on cytology nasal same as those found at the start of the study.
- **Increase:** Number of eosinophils in nasal cytology above the normal value.

L. Variables related to adverse reactions to sublingual immunotherapy. Qualitative Nominal:

Adverse reactions to immunotherapy are considered to be undesirable responses or harmful effects, intended or unintended, that occur when using a drug in the appropriate dose to obtain a therapeutic, prophylactic or diagnostic benefit, and depend on the characteristics of the individual, the product used, the route of administration, and the guidelines used.

In sublingual immunotherapy, adverse events are classified as local and systemic, the latter ranging from grade 0 to IV according to WAO:
Local reactions can be:

- **Mild:** oral or lingual itching, nausea, epigastralgia, which disappear spontaneously within 30 minutes, are relatively frequent and do not imply changes in the treatment regimen.
- **Moderate: they** last more than 30 minutes and require medication, which may be oral antihistamines, and a possible modification of the plan should be considered, reducing the dose to the immediate previous one.

Systemic reactions are considered:

▪ **Grade 0:** Presence of non-specific symptoms: headache, malaise, tiredness, arthralgia.
▪ **Grade I:** Mild focal events are considered, given by mild asthma and/or rhinitis, localised urticaria.
▪ **Grade II:** Focal adverse event of slow onset after 15 minutes, of moderate intensity, characterised by: moderate asthma and generalised urticaria, requires medication.

▪ **Grade III:** Severe non-life threatening focal event with rapid onset within 15 minutes, presenting with: severe asthma, angioedema, generalised urticaria, with immediate treatment to reverse the effect of the vaccine.
▪ **Grade IV:** Generalised systemic reaction, with immediate onset, characterised by pruritus, heat sensation, generalised erythema, generalised urticaria, stridor, severe asthma and arterial hypotension: anaphylactic shock.

In our study, adverse reactions were considered only in the study group, cases that received sublingual immunotherapy with mites, but not in the control group that only used pharmacological treatment, which was called:
▪ **Present:** Presence of local or systemic adverse reactions related to the administration of sublingual immunotherapy.
▪ **Absent:** No adverse reactions related to sublingual immunotherapy.

M. Variables related to the evolution of patients: Qualitative Nominal:
The author's criteria for the effectiveness of immunotherapy are assumed to include:
✓ 30% decrease in respiratory symptom score associated with bronchial asthma.
✓ No limitation in physical activity or mild limitation for those who were initially moderately to severely limited.
✓ Negative emergency visits.

✓ Behaviour of absences from work as good or non-absences.

✓ Normal or equal lung function.

✓ Does not use rescue medication.

✓ Saving of inhaled corticosteroids in section 3 and 4 (minimum dose or non-use).

✓ Immunoglobulin E levels considered adequate.

✓ Reduction in the number of nasal eosinophils.

✓ Absence of adverse reactions to sublingual immunotherapy.

Grouping into:

▪ **Favourable outcome:** Patients who met 6 or more of the established criteria for effectiveness.
▪ **Unfavourable outcome:** Patients with 5 or less established criteria for effectiveness.

Information processing:

Once the information was collected, it was processed in computerised form, for which a database was created on a Pentium IV computer using the statistical system SPSS version 11.5 for Windows for presentation in tables and graphs. Contingency or double-entry tables were constructed, summary measures were used for qualitative variables such as percentage and absolute numbers were used. To identify the statistically significant association, the Chi-square test of homogeneity was used, selecting a significance level of $\alpha = 0.05$. The results obtained were compared with other authors, conclusions and recommendations are made.

ANALYSIS AND DISCUSSION OF THE RESULTS

The prevalence of allergic diseases, including bronchial asthma, is increasing. It is estimated that more than 20% of the world's population suffers from IgE-mediated allergic diseases such as asthma, rhinoconjunctivitis, atopic dermatitis/eczema and anaphylaxis.[20-24, 42] Bronchial asthma is of allergic origin in more than 60% of adults and 80% of children and occurs in approximately 5-15% of the paediatric population,[45] causing an enormous health cost and is one of the main causes of hospitalisation for chronic disease, statistical data that have led various authors to call allergic diseases the "epidemic of the 21st century".[47-50]

Several studies have demonstrated the role of inhaled allergens in the exacerbation of allergic diseases, mainly bronchial asthma, both perennial (house dust mites, insects and animal shedding) and seasonal (pollens and fungi) allergens. Dust mites are among the most prevalent perennial allergens worldwide.[35-40, 42, 47]

Studies in Cuba show that mites of the genus Dermatophagoides and Glycyphagidae, particularly the species Dermatophagoides pteronyssinus, Dermatophagoides siboney and Blomia tropicalis, are of great importance as sensitising agents in allergic individuals.[43-48, 49]

One of the most frequent causes of respiratory allergies are faecal particles excreted by dust mites, which can become airborne and reach the respiratory tract, mainly found in dust accumulated in beds, mattresses, clothes, upholstered furniture and carpets.[41-48] Although genetic predisposition conditions susceptibility to respiratory allergic diseases, these diseases could not manifest themselves without exposure to environmental allergens.[49, 50]

For allergy sufferers, inhalers and a number of other specific medications are an important part of their life luggage, as these drugs accompany them wherever they go to avoid symptoms and overcome possible attacks.[11, 14-17] However, in recent decades, there is an alternative for many allergy sufferers that can lead to a significant improvement and even complete elimination of the disease.Immunotherapy opens a new avenue of treatment and solution for allergy sufferers and a new horizon for their ailments, considered as the specific treatment of allergic diseases that manages to modulate or modify the natural course of these pathologies.[25-30]

Several placebo-controlled studies have shown the efficacy and safety of this treatment, but further studies are needed to establish the place of sublingual immunotherapy in the treatment of allergic diseases. [23,26-29]Table 1 shows the distribution of patients according to age, with a predominance of patients aged 20-29 years with 13 patients for 29.5% and 29 for 33.3% for the study and control groups, the least predominant age group was 50-59 years with 7 patients for 16.0% and 15 patients for 17.0% respectively.

According to the Global Initiative for Asthma (GINA)[19] in February 2023 25% of adults in Great Britain, Australia and Canada suffer from some degree of bronchial asthma. Recent published studies show that the prevalence of the disease worldwide ranges from 1% to 30% in different latitudes; in Spain it is 4% to 20%, in the United States approximately 26 million people are affected; of these 8.6 million are under 18 years of age.

ISAAC (International Study of Asthma and Allergy in Childhood) studies carried out in our country show that by age, the prevalence of dispensed patients is 86 per 1,000 adults and 140 in children under 15 years of age.[5, 13-15, 61-65] The results obtained in our research are justified by the advances in the Cuban health system where the different levels of care are integrated, which has made possible the early diagnosis of these patients with the consequent increase in prevalence in age groups closer to paediatric age and old age. The need to plan intervention strategies from paediatric age is evident, since with adequate control from childhood, less morbidity is achieved in adulthood, according to Stone AH et al, as well as other authors.[20, 66,67]

Table 1. Distribution of persistent asthmatic patients and sublingual immunotherapy with mites according to age. Allergology Department. Saturnino Lora Provincial Hospital. January 2022 - 2024

GROUPS FROM AGES	STUDIO GROUP		CONTROL GROUP	
	No.	%	No.	%
From 20 to 29 years old	13	29.5	29	33.0
From 30 to 39 years old	13	29.5	28	31.8
From 40 to 49 years old	11	25.0	16	18.2
From 50 to 59 years old	7	16.0	15	17.0
TOTAL	44	100	88	100

Source: Data Collection Form.

When analysing Table 2 we observed that the female sex predominated with 28 patients for 63.6 % in the study group and 50 with 56.8 % in the control group, which represents more than half of the sample; the male sex was represented by 16 patients for 36.4 % and 38 with 43.2 % respectively.Similar results are reported in several studies in our country and internationally, such as the Global Initiative for Asthma (GINA),[19, 68, 69] which reports that bronchial asthma is more frequent in the male sex in a 2:1 ratio during childhood, but when puberty is reached, this ratio tends to equalise, with the female sex predominating in adulthood, and local studies such as Dr. Ferrer Alemán's residency thesis indicate that the female sex is the most frequent.[70] In a study conducted at the Clinical Immunology and Allergy Service of Mexico City by Velarde Domínguez and Talavera Hernández,[1] on the clinical efficacy and safety of sublingual immunotherapy in the treatment of allergic asthma, a predominance of the male sex was found in the sample studied, contrary to the results of our work.

Table 2. Distribution of persistent asthmatic patients and sublingual mite immunotherapy according to gender

STUDIO GROUP			CONTROL GROUP	
SEX	No.	%	No.	%
Female	28	63.6	50	56.8
Male	16	36.4	38	43.2
TOTAL	44	100	88	100

Table 3, which relates allergen sensitisation to skin reactivity in the study group, shows that more than half of the cases had negative skin reactivity, with monosensitised patients predominating, with a total of 39 patients (88.6 %). It is important to note that 22.7 % decreased reactivity, only 4 cases remained unchanged (9.1 %), and none of the monosensitised patients developed new sensitisation or increased pre-existing sensitisation.Only one polysensitised patient had reduced skin reactivity after treatment with sublingual immunotherapy, for 2.3%. Among the patients classified as bisensitised, we found 4 cases (9.1 %). %, 2 patients for 4.5 % were negative.In the selected study group no new sensitisations developed, regardless of the sensitivity found at the beginning of the investigation, revealing the reduction in skin reactivity related to the application of sublingual immunotherapy during two years of treatment to be statistically significant. Our casuistry was dominated by patients monosensitised by the Dermatophagoides pteronyssinus mite, coinciding with the work carried out by Dr Mayda González León, Dr Raúl Lázaro Castro, Mirtha Álvarez Castelló, Dr Alexis Labrada Rosado and collaborators,[21] in a health area of La Lisa, Havana City and in the coastal area of our capital. In Latin America, sensitisation to different mite species has been frequently reported in a study by Martinez et al. who demonstrated a sensitisation prevalence of more than 75 % for 4 mite species (D. siboney, D. pteronyssinus, Acarus siro and Blomia tropicalis). Maldonado Pérez, et. al.[34] believe that it would be interesting and useful to typify allergic sensitisation in patients with asthma and rhinitis, preferably measured by prick test, which is necessary for better clinical and epidemiological control. We found similarities with the results obtained in research carried out in Mexico by

Olimpo Rodríguez, Pérez Martin and Martínez Jiménez, et al.[11, 12, 15, 68, 69]

Distribution of persistent asthma patients and sublingual immunotherapy according to allergen sensitisation and skin reactivity.

Awareness-raising	Sensitised Monkey		Bi-sensitised		Sensitised poly		Total	
	No.	%	No.	%	No.	%	No.	%
Negative Reactivity	25	56.8	2	4.5	0	0	27	61.3
Decreased Reactivity	10	22.7	1	2.3	1	2.3	12	27.3
Reactivity Equal	4	9.1	1	2.3	0	0	5	11.4
New Awareness	0	0	0	0	0	0	0	0
Total	39	88.6	4	9.1	1	2.3	44	100

p< 0,05

In table 4, which shows the symptomatology of the patients stratified by levels, depending on the appearance of bronchial obstruction and allergic respiratory syndrome symptoms during the day or at night, taking into consideration the frequency of their variation over the course of the month, we found that at the beginning of the study, in both groups, patients with daytime symptoms more than once a week and night-time symptoms more than twice a month predominated (level 2), with 18 patients (40.9 %) in the study group and 32 patients (36.4 %) in the control group, followed by cases in level 3 (29.5 %) and 32 patients (36.4 %) in the control group, followed by cases in level 3 (29.5 %) and 32 patients (36.4 %).9 % in the study group and 32 patients representing 36.4 % in the control group, followed by the cases in level 3, with 29.5 and 23.9 % respectively.With daily nocturnal and diurnal symptoms (level 4) we had at the beginning of the study only 5 patients in the study group for 11.4 %, and 11 in the control group for 12.5 %. When evaluating the casuistry two years a f t e r treatment with immunotherapy we found that in the study group no patients remained in level 4; only 2 cases were in level 3 for 4.5 %, 15 in level 2 for 34.1 %, and the majority were in level 1 with 27 cases for 61.4 %.However, when we reviewed the control group we found that 36 patients were in level 1 for 40.9 %, but a non-negligible group of asthmatics remained in levels 3 and 4, with frequent daytime and night-time symptoms, with 17 patients in the third level for 19.3 % and 8 for 9.1 % in the fourth level. Statistical analysis showed that the results were statistically significant in relation to the symptomatology presented.

When comparing the results obtained in our research with other efficacy studies carried out by various authors, we found similarities in terms of the reduction in the symptom score presented by asthmatic patients who received sublingual immunotherapy. Abramson and collaborators (1995 and 1999) concluded that patients who had received immunotherapy presented fewer asthma symptoms and were less likely to have their disease deteriorate, so that the vaccines were more effective in reducing asthma symptoms. Anti-allergic agents are a valid option for the treatment of patients with allergic asthma.[5-11]

Ross and colleagues also published a new meta-analysis on the effectiveness of allergen immunotherapy in asthma, where the authors confirmed that in the immunotherapy-treated group there was a reduction of symptom markers.[8, 9, 12]

Maurizio Marogna et al,[25] last year published a 15-year study on sublingual immunotherapy in bronchial asthma, concluding that it has many short- and long-term benefits, including a significant reduction in symptom score, Velarde Domínguez and collaborators[1] found similar effects with regard to the reduction of asthmatic symptomatology with sublingual immunotherapy with mites, results that coincide with those of our research.

Distribution of persistent asthma patients and sublingual mite immunotherapy according to symptomatology.

STUDIO GROUP				CONTROL GROUP			
Symptoms	NO HOME	%	1 YEAR	NO HOME	%	1 YEAR	
Level 1	8	18.2	27	61.4	24	27.2	36	40.9
Level 2	18	40.9	15	34.1	32	36.4	27	30.7
Level 3	13	29.5	2	4.5	21	23.9	17	19.3
Level 4	5	11.4	0	0	11	12.5	8	9.1
Total	44	100	44	100	88	100	88	100

p< 0,05

In Table 5, when considering the limitation of activities, initially 15 patients presented moderate limitation, for 34.1 % and 8 cases presented severe limitation for 18.2 %; in the control group initially the asthmatics with slight limitation predominated with 32 patients for 36.4 %, followed by those with moderate limitation with 27 for 30.6 %, without limitation 16 patients representing 18.2 % with only 3 cases less. without activity limitations. During two years of treatment in the study group we found that only 2 patients remained without physical activity for 4.5 %, increasing to 18 with slight limitations for 40.9 %, leaving 17 cases without limitations to physical activities for 38.6 %. In the control group, the number of cases with moderate limitations was reduced to 19 for 21.6 %, while those with slight limitations increased to 38 for 43.2 % and those with no limitations to 24 for 27.3 %. We found no statistically significant differences in the two groups. Compared to the literature, studies such as those by Muñoz López and Pedemonte Marco in Spain,[26] show that physical exercise is not modified in the short term (less than three years of treatment) with sublingual immunotherapy, and this is related to the limited improvement in lung function that is produced; we found similar effects in our research.

Table 5. Distribution of persistent asthma patients and sublingual mite immunotherapy according to activity limitation.

STUDIO GROUP					CONTROL GROUP		
Limitation of activities	NO HOME	% 1 YEAR			NO HOME	% 1 YEAR	
No limitation	11	25.0	17	38.6	16	18.2	24	27.3
Slight limitation	10	22.7	18	40.9	32	36.4	38	43.2
Moderate limitation	15	34.1	7	16.0	27	30.6	19	21.6
Severe limitation	8	18.2	2	4.5	13	14.8	7	7.9
TOTAL	44	100	44	100	88	100	88	100

$p > 0.05$

Table 6 shows the number of visits to the emergency department by asthmatic patients. When analysing the study group, we see that at the beginning 19 patients did not attend the emergency department (43.2 %), a figure that almost doubles one year after treatment with sublingual immunotherapy, with 35 patients (79.5 %); The slightly positive group decreased by half, from 14 at baseline to 7 at one year representing 16.0 %, in the strongly positive group from 4 cases at baseline to 9.0 %, no patients remained with more than seven emergency room visits and admissions, which speaks for better control of the disease, and less deterioration of these patients as a whole. In the control group of 19 patients who started the study as strong positives, after one year with environmental and pharmacological control treatment this was reduced to 12 cases for 13.6 %, in the median positive there was no significant reduction, only one case left the group, we consider that the control group showed little variation in terms of visits to the emergency department of persistent asthmatic patients. The relationship with visits to the emergency department and sublingual immunotherapy was statistically significant with p < 0.05. On consulting the literature on the subject, Muñoz López and Pedemonte Marco,[26] agree with our results, stating that immunotherapy has been shown to be beneficial in preventing deterioration of the disease, as it reduces symptoms, use of medication and therefore admissions to the emergency department. Thus studies by César Martín Bózzola,[27] in Buenos Aires, Argentina make references to the reduction in the number of hospitalisations in persistent asthma patients receiving sublingual immunotherapy, similar to those found in our research. Summarising the Global Strategy for Asthma Management and Prevention (GINA),[19] defines asthma as a serious public health problem throughout the world, affecting people of all ages. When asthma is uncontrolled, it can place severe limits on daily life, and is sometimes fatal.

Table 6. Distribution of persistent asthma patients and sublingual mite immunotherapy according to number of visits to the emergency department.

STUDIO GROUP				CONTROL GROUP			
Emergency visits	NO HOME	% 1 YEAR		NO HOME	% 1 YEAR		
Negative	19	43.2	35	79.5	26	29.5	31	35.2
Slightly positive	14	31.8	7	16.0	25	28.4	28	31.9
Positive medium	7	16.0	2	4.5	18	20.5	17	19.3
Strong positive	4	9.0	0	0	19	21.6	12	13.6
TOTAL	44	100	44	100	88	100	88	100

$p < 0.05$

Table 7 shows the distribution of patients according to absenteeism from work, finding in the case studies of our study group that at the beginning 33 patients (75.0 %) had no absenteeism from work, two years after receiving the allergen extract sublingually, except for 2 patients (4.5 %). This is an important variable when taking into account the quality of life of the patients, since financial remuneration is essential to cover individual needs; moreover, the health costs generated by chronic non-communicable diseases are not negligible. In the control group the difference at the beginning of treatment and at two years was 10 cases, 52 for 59.1 %, and at two years 62 asthmatic patients without absenteeism, which represented 70.5 %, but 26 remained for 29.5 % with 5 or more absences from work. Statistically significant results were obtained for this variable in both groups. In consulting the literature on the subject, the World Health Organisation,[19]has estimated that 15 million disability-adjusted life years (DALYs) are lost annually due to asthma, representing 1% of the total global burden of disease. Social and economic factors must be integrated to understand asthma and its management, whether viewed from the perspective of the perspective of the individual sufferer, the health care professional, or the organisations that pay for health care. Days lost from work are reported as a major social and economic problem of asthma in studies in India, the Asia-Pacific region, the United States and the United Kingdom, India and Latin America. Asthma is the most frequent cause of absenteeism from work in Australia, Sweden, the United Kingdom and the United States. [28, 29, 30]

Distribution of persistent asthmatic patients according to absenteeism from work.

STUDIO GROUP				CONTROL GROUP			
Absenteeism Labour	NO HOME	% 1 YEAR		NO HOME		% 1 YEAR	
ABSENT	33	75.0	42	95.5	52	59.1	62	70.5
PRESENT	11	25.0	2	4.5	36	40.9	26	29.5
TOTAL	44	100	44	100	88	100	88	100

p< 0.05

Table 8 shows the variations of lung function in the patients studied initially 9 cases 20.4 % had worsened lung function, of which 3 improved and remained in the group 6 asthmatic patients with FEV1/FVC ratio less than 75 %; with normal function 19 cases at baseline for 43.2 %, 5 cases belonging to the other groups recovered, i.e. improved lung function for 24 asthmatics with normal lung function, representing 54.5 %, there were no cases with worsened lung function.In the control group, the behaviour was similar, with little variability in the number of patients with improved lung function, but of greater significance were the cases with worsened lung function: of 18 (20.5 %) initially, 12 cases remained for a total of 13.6 %. When the Chi-square test was applied to the lung function variable, it was not statistically significant (p > 0.05).Compared to other research, we do not agree with the results obtained by Ross and colleagues, who published a meta-analysis of the results of their research. analysis of the effectiveness of allergen immunotherapy in asthma, where the authors confirmed that the immunotherapy group acquired protection against bronchial challenge and improved lung function. [66] Similar results to ours were obtained in meta-analyses by Abramson et al. (1995, 1999, 2003),[5, 6, 7]

Malling,[63, 64] in 1998 and Bousquet,[69] in 1998, which showed that immunotherapy did not significantly improve lung function and specific bronchial hyperresponsiveness.[34]

Table 8. Distribution of persistent asthma patients and sublingual immunotherapy by lung function

STUDIO GROUP				CONTROL GROUP			
Lung function	NO HOME	% 1 YEAR	NO HOME	% 1 YEAR			
Normal	19	43.2	24	54.5	32	36.3	35	39.8
Equal	16	36.4	14	31.8	38	43.2	41	16.6
Worsened	9	20.4	6	13.6	18	20.5	12	13.6
TOTAL	44	100	44	100	88	100	88	100

p> 0.05

When analysing Table 9 we found that initially in the study group all patients used rescue medication, two years after treatment only 7 patients remained in this group, for 15.9 %, and more than one third of the sample did not use rescue medication, for a total of 37 asthmatics, which constitutes 84.1 %.

In the control group, initially 100 % of the patients used rescue medication, during the two years of pharmacological treatment approximately half of the cases were distributed in both categories, with 47 asthmatics remaining for 53.4 % using rescue medication, obtaining statistically significant results at p < 0.05.

When comparing the results with those obtained by other authors, we find a coincidence, as Muñoz López and Pedemonte Marco,[2] point out A significant decrease in the use of relief medication in those individuals who received immunotherapy with mites and pollens than in those who received placebo, and those who were treated with the active ingredient had less need to increase the medication they were taking as a base. Other studies such as those by Lorente Toledano, Laffond, Moreno and Dávila,[67] in Salamanca, Spain, reveal significant reductions in medication requirements during and after immunotherapy treatment.

Table 9. Distribution of persistent asthma patients and sublingual immunotherapy according to use of rescue medication

STUDIO GROUP				CONTROL GROUP			
Rescue medication	NO START	% 1 YEAR		NO START	% 1 YEAR		
Does not use	0	0	37	84.1	0	0	41	46.6
Use	44	100	7	15.9	88	100	47	53.4
TOTAL	44	100	44	100	88	100	88	100

$$p < 0.05$$

When analysing table 10 showing the distribution of patients according to inhaled corticosteroid sparing, we see in the study group that the majority of patients were located in section 3, with 28 cases using the minimum dose of fluticasone for 63.6% and 4 asthmatics using the maximum dose of the same, for 9.1%, only 7 patients (15.9%) did not use inhaled steroids as a controller treatment for Bronchial Asthma.Two years after treatment with sublingual mite immunotherapy, only 2 patients remained in sections 1 and 2, with high doses of inhaled steroids, for 2.3 %; the majority of our cases were in section 4, without the use of controller medication, 37 cases for 84.0 %.In the control group however, in section 4, from 18 patients initially (20.5 %) it increased to 23 (26.1 %), recovering only 5 cases that did not use fluticasone spray, in this group there was no increase in cases with maximum dose of medication, 11 (12.5 %) at the beginning and at one year 5 cases for5.7%. When applying the statistical significance test, we obtained statistically significant results.Comparatively, studies have shown that sublingual immunotherapy is also used in other parts of the world, such as Asia, and in July 2010 the results of a Phase I clinical study were published. III in China that has demonstrated the efficacy and safety of sublingual allergen immunotherapy (Staloral® 300)[3] in adults with house dust mite asthma.Similar studies have been published by Ross and colleagues who reported a reduction in markers of asthma symptoms and drug use.[66] Coinciding with these results we can cite other authors such as Abramson and colleagues,[5, 6, 7] Wilson DR, Torres Lima and Durham,[13, 14] Maurizio Marogna and colleagues.[25]

Table 10. Distribution of persistent asthmatic patients and sublingual immunotherapy according to inhaled corticosteroid sparing

STUDIO GROUP				CONTROL GROUP			
Saving corticosteroids	NO START	% 1 YEAR		NO START	% 1 YEAR		
Paragraph 1	4	9.1	1	2.3	11	12.5	5	5.7
Paragraph 2	5	11.4	1	2.3	23	26.1	15	17.1
Paragraph 3	28	63.6	5	11.4	36	40.9	45	51.1
Paragraph 4	7	15.9	37	84.0	18	20.5	23	26.1
TOTAL	44	100	44	100	88	100	88	100

p < 0.05

Table 11 shows the distribution of patients according to immunoglobulin E levels, in the study group initially 24 of the patients had adequate levels of the antibody for 54.5 %, and 20 cases (45.5 %) had adequate levels of immunoglobulin E for 54.5 %, and 20 cases (45.5 %) had inadequate levels of immunoglobulin E for 54.5 %.At one year after treatment, only two cases joined the group with adequate immunoglobulin E levels, with 26 patients (59.1%) and 18 patients with inadequate levels (40.9%).In the control group, the behaviour of this variable is very similar to the study group, with little variability in the start and year of pharmacological treatment. Chi-square analysis was not statistically significant.

When we compare the results obtained with the bibliography consulted, we observe that the levels of antibodies and specifically immunoglobulin E, do not change in the short term with sublingual immunotherapy but with treatments lasting more than three years, thus we can cite Maldonado and collaborators34 , César Martín Bózzola27 , Wurcel V.24 and other authors, who coincide with our results, from our point of view in our study these results correspond to the short time that the therapeutic alternative was used.

Table 11. Distribution of persistent asthmatic patients and sublingual immunotherapy according to IgE levels

STUDIO GROUP				CONTROL GROUP			
IgE levels	NO HOME	% 1 YEAR		NO HOME	% 1 YEAR		
Adequate	24	54.5	26	59.1	49	55.6	46	52.3
Inadequate	20	45.5	18	40.9	39	44.4	42	47.7
TOTAL	44	100	44	100	88	100	88	100

p > 0.05

In table 12 we relate the nasal eosinophils as an indicator of the local inflammatory response, we obtained that at the beginning of the study most of the cases were located in the group with an increase in the number of nasal eosinophils for 23 patients which represented 52.3 %, after 24 months receiving sublingual immunotherapy only 1 patient remained in this group for 2.3 %, rising to 40 cases that presented reduction in the number of eosinophils, for 90.9 %.In the control group there was a decrease in nasal eosinophil numbers, but less significant, so that from 21 cases (23.8 %) at the beginning of the investigation, 30 patients were added to the group with normal nasal cytology eosinophil numbers or with a reduction in the percentage found at the beginning of the investigation.of the study, 15 patients remained with increased nasal eosinophils for 17.1 %. The result was statistically significant for both groups. Inflammation in the asthmatic patient is considered to remain a constant feature and affects all airways including the nose (GINA),[19]and therefore we consider it of vital importance to evaluate the behaviour of eosinophil counts by nasal smear in our study.Studies by Abramson, Puy and Weiner,[6] in 2008 show similar results to those obtained in our study, with a significant reduction in nasal eosinophils. Studies measuring inflammatory response parameters in patients undergoing sublingual immunotherapy have been carried out by Muñoz López and Pedemonte Marco,[21] who found that there was no change in nasal eosinophilia but there was a decrease in nasal and bronchial symptoms in the groups studied, which does not coincide with the results obtained in our study.

Table 12. Distribution of persistent asthma patients and sublingual immunotherapy according to local inflammatory response mediated by nasal eosinophils.

STUDIO GROUP				CONTROL GROUP			
Nasal eosinophils	NO START	% 1 YEAR		NO START		% 1 YEAR	
Reduction	10	22.7	40	90.9	21	23.8	51	57.9
Maintenance	11	25.0	3	6.8	20	22.7	22	25.0
Increase	23	52.3	1	2.3	47	53.5	15	17.1
TOTAL	44	100	44	100	88	100	88	100

$p < 0.05$

Table 13 shows the adverse reactions to sublingual immunotherapy that occurred during the course of the research in the study group; these occurred in only 4 cases for 9.1 %, these were mild local adverse reactions, given by three cases with pruritus. The oral administration and one case of nausea disappeared spontaneously within 30 minutes, and did not require changes in the treatment regimen. There were no systemic adverse reactions. The result was statistically significant at $p < 0.05$. Similar results have been published by several authors, who report few adverse reactions with the application of sublingual immunotherapy; there are no studies reporting systemic adverse reactions in this treatment variant. Research by Velarde Domínguez and Talavera Hernández,[1, 3, 4] Maurizio Marogna, Muñoz López and Pedemonte Marco, and others are related.[23-26, 44-47]

Table 13. Distribution of persistent asthma patients and sublingual immunotherapy according to Adverse Reactions.

Adverse reactions	No.	%
PRESENTS	4	9.1
ABSENT	40	90.9
TOTAL	44	100

$p < 0.05$

Table 14 shows the final evolution of the patients: in the study group, 30 patients evolved favourably (68.2 %) and in the control group 32 cases (36.4 %); with an unfavourable evolution in the study group we found 14 cases that did not meet 6 or more of the established criteria for effectiveness, and in the control group more than half of them (68.2 %). 63.6 % showed an unfavourable evolution. Statistically significant results. On consulting the literature, we found that in several meta-analyses and double-blind, placebo-controlled studies the results have been similar, concluding that sublingual immunotherapy is an effective alternative in the treatment of bronchial asthma, due to the short and long-term benefits obtained with it; effects emanate in the decrease of controller medication and exacerbations, decrease in asthmatic symptoms score, fewer exacerbations, with decrease in absences. The treatment is considered an effective, feasible treatment that modifies the natural course of allergic diseases.23-27, 34, 40, 44, 46, 47, 50-53, 58

Table 14. Distribution of persistent asthmatic patients and sublingual immunotherapy according to the evolution of the patients

Evolution of the patients	Study Group		Control Group	
	No.	%	No.	%
Favourable	30	68.2	32	36.4
Unfavourable	14	31.8	56	63.6
Total	44	100	88	100

p < 0.05

The results of our research substantiate that sublingual immunotherapy has represented an alternative for the follow-up and control of asthmatic patients, emerging as the best option in view of the persistence of clinical benefit; some fifteen years ago there were only few data on its lasting effect.Today, thanks to science, there is other evidence that makes us consider it as a powerful tool for tackling one of the diseases that, due to its worldwide prevalence, represents a real challenge for medical science. Achieving timely control that ensures quality of life in accordance with the changing needs of a world besieged by various conflicts motivates us to continue to study it in depth.

CONCLUSIONS

The research identified favourable variations in the effectiveness of allergen-specific sublingual immunotherapy with mites in mild and moderate persistent asthma patients during two years of treatment, which resulted in reduced symptoms, fewer visits to the emergency department, less use of rescue and controller medication, and only local adverse reactions, which positively influenced the control and improvement of the quality of life of these patients.

RECOMMENDATIONS

Continuing research to identify variations in the long-term effectiveness of immunotherapy.

BIBLIOGRAPHICAL REFERENCES

Velarde Domínguez T, Talavera Hernández O, Sánchez Santa AJ, Madrigal Mendoza LF. Clinical efficacy and safety of sublingual immunotherapy with standardised extracts in the treatment of allergic asthma caused by dermatophagoides in a Mexican paediatric population. Alergología Viltual [online document] 2001 [cited January 2024]; Available from:
http://www.alergovirtual.org.ar/trabajoslibres/23.htm/2001/01/15/

2. - Hankin CS, Cox L, Lang D, Levin A, Gross G, Eavy G, Meltzer E, Burgoyne D, Bronstone A, Wang Z. Allergy immunotherapy among Medicaid-enrolled children with allegic rhinitis: Patterns of care, resource use, and costs. J Allergy Clin Immunol [article on the Internet] 2008 [cited January 2024]; 121: 227-32. Available from:
https://pubmed.ncbi.nlm.nih.gov/18206509/

3.-Pepys J. Atopy, In: Gill P, Coombs RRA, Lachman PJ (eds) Clinical aspects of immunology [article on the Internet] 1975 [cited January 2024]; 8887-902 Blackwell Scientific. Available from:
https://www.seaic.org/wp-content/uploads/2019/07/gell_coombs_clinical_immunology_1968_seaic.pdf

4.-Abramson MJ, Puy R M, Weiner JM. Is allergen specific immunotherapy effective in asthma. A meta-analysis of randomized controlled trials. Am J Respir Care Med [article on the Internet] 1995 [cited January 2024]; 151:969- 974. Available from:
https://pubmed.ncbi.nlm.nih.gov/7697274/

Abramson M J, Puy RM, Weiner JM. Allergen specific immunotherapy for asthma. In the Cochrane Lybrary Review; issue 4: [online book] 2010 [cited on January from 2024]; Oxford. Available at:
https://www.cochranelibrary.com/cdsr/doi/10.1002/14651858.CD001186.pub2/a bstract

Ishizaka K, Ishizaka T. Identification of gamma-E antibodies as carrier of reaginic antibody. J Immunol [article on the Internet] 1967 [cited January 2024]; 99:1187. Available from:
https://pubmed.ncbi.nlm.nih.gov/4168663/

7.-Águila de la Coba R. History of immunotherapy in Cuba. [Varadero 18 - 22 April 2009]. Congreso Internacional Cuba Alergia 2009. [cited

January 2024]. Available from: https://uvscuba.sld.cu/detalles-del-resource/eventos/1022

8.-Pérez PML, García DA, Sabina DA, Vega GM, Macías CV. Sensitization to different types of mites in adult patients. Rev. Cubana Med.

Internet] 2002 [cited January 2024]; 41(2): 75-8. Available from: http://scielo.sld.cu/scielo.php?script=sci_arttext&pid=S0034-75232002000200002

9.-Duce Gracia DF. Epicutaneous tests for the diagnosis of allergy. Atlas of Allergy and Clinical Immunology. [online document] 2000 [cited January 2024]; VIII: 101-105. Available from: https://www.cun.es/enfermedades- tratamientos/pruebas-diagnosticas/pruebas-alergia-cutaneas.

10.- Rodríguez SO. Sublingual immunotherapy in rhinitisallergicrhinitisasthma in children aged 2-5 years sensitized to mites. Rev. Allerg. Mexico. [article on the Internet] 2008 [cited January 2024];55(2):71-75. Available from: http://scielo.sld.cu/scielo.php?script=sci_arttext&pid=S1025-028X2015000200005

11.- Rodríguez Santos O, Rodríguez VM. Bronchial asthma in children. Sublingual immunotherapy with Dermatophagoides pteronyssinus as a treatment alternative. Ciencia Pediatrika. 2005; 25(6):18-21. Available at: https://pesquisa.bvsalud.org/portal/resource/pt/ibc-041195

12.-Wilson DR, Torres Lima M, Durham SR. Sublingual immunotherapy for allergic rhinitis. In: The Cochrane Library, Issue 3, [document online] 2010 [cited January 2024]. Oxford: Update Software. Available in: https://www.cochranelibrary.com/cdsr/doi/10.1002/14651858.CD002893.pub2/a bstract

Wilson DR, Torres Lima M, Durham SR. Sublingual immunotherapy for allergic rhinitis. In: The Cochrane Library Plus, Issue 4, [online document] 2006 [cited January 2024]; Oxford. Available from: https://www.cochranelibrary.com/es/

14.-Risci CD, Ardusso LRF. Prevalence of aeroallergen sensitivity in Cordoba. Arch Arg Allergia Inmunol Clin [article on the Internet] 2003 [cited in January from 2024];23(4):32-44.Available en: http://scielo.sld.cu/scielo.php?script=sci_arttext&pid=S1025-02552004000100008

15.-Lund L, Henmar H, Würtzen PA, Lund G, Hjortskov N, Larsen JN.

Comparison of allergenicity and immunogenic of an intact allergen vaccine and commercially available allergoid products for birch pollen immunotherapy. Clin

Exp Allergy. [article on the Internet] 2007 [cited January 2024]; 37(4):56471. Available from: https://pubmed.ncbi.nlm.nih.gov/17430354/

16.-O'Hehir RE, Sandrini A, Anderson GP, Rolland JM. Sublingual allergen immunotherapy: immunological mechanisms and prospects for refined vaccine preparation. Curr Med Chem. [article on the Internet] 2007 [cited January 2024]. 14(21):223544.Available at: https://pubmed.ncbi.nlm.nih.gov/17896972/

17.-Allergic Diseases: Epidemiology and Allergy March. [document on line] 2007 [cited on January 2024]; Available from: http://www.scai.cl//

18.-Gina: Global strategy for the management and prevention of asthma. [Ontario; 2006:77-8. [Cited: 26 Dec 2010]. Available from: http://www.ginasthama.org.

19.-Stone AH, García CR, López GA, Barragán MM, Sánchez CG. Childhood Asthma: Guidelines for diagnosis and treatment. [document online] 2005 [cited January 2024];14(1) 2005; 18-36. Available from: https://www.medigraphic.com/pdfs/alergia/al-2005/al051d.pdf

20.-Muñoz LF, Pedemonte MC.Immunotherapy: Mechanisms of action, indications and benefits. Diagnostic and therapeutic protocols in Paediatrics. Clinical Immunol. and Allerg. [article on the Internet] 2005 [cited January 2024];12(6);127-135. Available at: https://www.aeped.es/sites/default/files/documentos/06_inmunoterapia_es pecifi ca.pdf

Castro AR, Álvarez CM, Ronquillo DM, Rodríguez CJ, García GI, González LM, Enríquez DI, Labrada RA et al. Sensitization to three mite species in allergic patients in the coastal area of the city of Havana. Revista Alergia México [article on the Internet] 2009 [cited January 2024]; 56(2):31-35.Available at: https://www.researchgate.net/publication/239579191_Sensibilizacion_a_tr es_es pecies_of_mite_in_allergic_patients_in_the_coastal_area_of_the_city Havana

22.-Bedolla BM, Hernández CD. Sensitization to aeroallergens in subjects with allergic rhinitis living in the metropolitan area of Guadalajara, Mexico. Revista Alergia México [article on the Internet]

2010 [cited in January 2010].

2024];57(2):50-56. Available at:
https://www.revistaalergia.mx/ojs/index.php/ram/article/view/634/1189

23.-Frew AJ. Sublingual immunotherapy. N Engl J Med. [article on the Internet] 2008 [cited January 2024]; May 22; 358(21):2259-64. Available from: https://www.nejm.org/doi/full/10.1056/NEJMct0708337

24.-Wurcel V. Efficacy and safety of immunotherapy in the treatment of asthma and allergy. Current Ambulatory Evid. [article on the Internet] 2004 [cited on January from 2024];7:186-187. Available available at: https://pesquisa.bvsalud.org/portal/resource/pt/lil-516188

Marogna M, et al. Sublingual immunotherapy for asthma and allergic rhinitis. JACI [article on the Internet] 2010 [cited January 2024]; 126:969-75. Available in:
https://flaviomaticorena.wordpress.com/2011/01/25/inmunoterapia-sublingual- para-asthma-and-allergic-rhinitis/

26.- Muñoz López C. Pedemonte Marco. Inmunotherapy: mechanisms of action, indications and benefits: Clinical immunology and allergology. Diagnostic and therapeutic protocols in paediatrics. [document online] 2006 [cited in January 2024]; 12: 127- 136. Available at: https://dialnet.unirioja.es/servlet/libro?codigo=942586

27.- César Martín Bózzola. Immunotherapy of allergic diseases in Paediatrics. Archivos de Alergia e Inmunología Clínica. [article on the Internet] 2004 [cited at January from 2024]; 35; 1:5-10. Available at: https://www.researchgate.net/publication/270592172_Inmunoterapia_de_l as_en
fermedades_alergicas_en_Pediatria_In_immunotherapy_in_pediatric_alle rgic_diseases_dise ases

Weinstein MC, Stason WB. Foundations of cost-effectiveness analysis for health and medical practices. N Engl J Med [article on the Internet] 1977 [cited January 2024];296 (13):716-21. Available from: https://pubmed.ncbi.nlm.nih.gov/402576/

Weiss KB, Sullivan SD. The economic costs of asthma: a review and conceptual model. Pharmacoeconomics [article in Internet] 1993 [cited in January from 2024];4 (1):14-30. Available at: https://pubmed.ncbi.nlm.nih.gov/10146965/

Carrol L. Action asthma: the occurrence and cost of asthma. West Sussex, United Kingdom: Cambridge Medical Publications; [document online] 1990. [cited 2024 January 2024] Available from:

https://www.immunology.theclinics.com/article/S0889-8561(05)70276-9/abstract 31.-Novak N, Bieber T, Allam J-P. Immunological mechanisms of sublingual allergen-specific immunotherapy. Allergy [article on the Internet] 2011 [cited January 2024]; Available from: https://doi.10.1111/j.1398-9995.2010.02535.

32.-Novak N, Haberstok J, Bieber T, Allam JP. The immune privilege of the oral mucosa. Trends Mol Med [article on the Internet] 2008 [cited January 2024];14: 191-198. Available at: https://pubmed.ncbi.nlm.nih.gov/18396104/ 33.- Herrera Suárez A, Carreño Rolando IE, Camacho Sosa K, Santiesteban Álvarez E, Morales Fuentes MA. Santos. History and indications of immunotherapy.Salud pública. [document online] 2007 [cited January 2024]; 49: 218-321. Available at: https://revmedicaelectronica.sld.cu/index.php/rme/article/view/3234/html_701 34.-Maldonado Pérez JA, et al. Inmunotherapy and asthma. Neumosur [article on the Internet] 2006 [cited January 2024]; 18, 4: 212-224. Available from: https://www.rev-esp-patol-torac.com/files/publicaciones/Revistas/2006/NS2006.18.4.A05.pdf

35.-Rodríguez AA, Cué MB. Behaviour of bronchial asthma in Cuba and importance of the prevention of allergic diseases in infants. Rev. Cubana Med. Integr [article on the Internet] 2006 [cited January 2024]; 22 (1). Available en: http://scielo.sld.cu/scielo.php?script=sci_arttext&pid=S0864-21252006000100013

Lyons AS, Petrucelli RJ. History of Medicine. [book online] 1987 [cited January from 2024]; Barcelona: Ediciones Doyma. Available at: https://www.iberlibro.com/buscar-libro/titulo/historia-de-la-medicina/autor/lyons- albert-s-petrucelli-joseph/

37.-Sánchez de la Vega W, Sánchez de la Vega E. From Clinical Allergy to Molecular Allergology: A concise 100-year history. Archives of Allergy and Clinical Immunology. [article on the Internet] 2007 [cited January 2024]; 38(3): 91-106.Available from: http://adm.meducatium.com.ar/contenido/articulos/9400910106_620/pdf/9 4009 10106.pdf

38.-Díaz RA, Fabré ODE, Coutin MG, Gonzáles MT. Sensitization to mites. Relationship with atopic diseases in schoolchildren in San Antonio de los Baños. Rev. Alerg. Mex. [article on the Internet] 2009 [cited January 2024]; 56(3):80-5. Available available at:

https://www.researchgate.net/publication/267260571_Sensibilizacion_a_a caros
Relationship_with_atopic_diseases_in_schools_in_San_Antonio_de_lo_s _Banos

39.-Talesnik GE, Hoyos BR. New nomenclature of allergic diseases. Its application to paediatric practice. Revista chilena de pediatría. [article on the Internet] 2006 [cited January 2024]; 77 (3); 239-46. Available from: http://www.scielo.cl/scielo.php?script=sci_arttext&pid=S0370-41062006000300002

Labrada Rosado A. Development of the first standardized mite allergen vaccines for asthma immunotherapy in Cuba. [Thesis on line]. Work for the scientific degree of Dr. in Health Sciences. Havana; 2008. [Cited: 18 Jan 2011]. Available at: http://tesis.repo.sld.cu/145.

41.-González M, Castro RL, Labrada A, Navarro B, Álvarez M, García I. Prevalence of sensitization to three house dust mites in the allergic infant population of a medical office in Havana City, Jan-Apr. 2005. Rev Cubana Med Gen Integr [article on the Internet] 2005 [cited January 2024];21(1-2). Available from: http://www.infomed.cu

42.- Negrín Villavicencio JA. Asma Bronquial, Aspectos básicos para un tratamiento integral según etapa clínica. Havana: Editorial Ciencias Médicas; [book online] 2004 [cited January 2024]; 1:1. Available from: http://www.ecimed.sld.cu/2004/12/01/asma-bronquial-aspectos-basicos-para- un-tratamiento-integral-segun-la-etapa-clinica-primera-edicion/

43.-Dávila HJ, Alfaro CJ, Brenes DA. Guías para la detección diagnóstico y tratamiento del asma bronquial en la edad adulta y adulta mayor en el primer nivel de atención. San José, Costa Rica. Caja Costarricense del seguro social; [article on the Internet] 2006 [cited January 2024]; (1-12) 5-17. Available from: https://www.binasss.sa.cr/protocolos/asma.pdf

44.-Hernández UF, Castillo GJ, Cabello RF, Ayerbe GR, Sánchez Armengol MA, Ortega Ruíz F. Immunotherapy in bronchial asthma sensitive to mites. Efficacy study. Neumosur [article on the Internet] 1993. [cited January 2024];vol.5, (2); September. Available at: https://dialnet.unirioja.es/servlet/articulo?codigo=7419617

45.-Lockey RF, Nicoara-Kasti GL, Theodoropoulos DS, Bukantz SC. Systemic reactions and fatalities associated with allergen immunotherapy. Ann Allergy Asthma Immunol [article on the Internet] 2001 [cited January 2024], 87(suppl 1):47-55. Available from:

https://pubmed.ncbi.nlm.nih.gov/11476476/
46.-Canonica GW, Passalacqua G. Noninjection routes for immunotherapy. J Allergy Clin Immunol [article on the Internet] 2003 [cited January 2024], 111:437-48. PubMed Abstract.at: https://pubmed.ncbi.nlm.nih.gov/12642818/
47.-Wilson DR, Torres-Lima M, Durham S: Sublingual immunotherapy for allergic rhinitis: systematic review and meta-analysis. Allergy 2005, 60:4-12.
48.-Shekelle PG, Woolf SH, Eccles M, Grimshaw J: Clinical guidelines: developing guidelines. BMJ 1999, 318:593-96.
49.-Wilson D, Torres-Lima M, Durham S: Sublingual immunotherapy for allergic rhinitis. Cochrane Database of Systematic Reviews [article on the Internet] 2003 [cited January 2024],(2):CD002893. Available from: https://doi.10.1002/14651858.CD002893
50.-Sopo SM, Macchiaolo M, Zorzi G, Tripodi S. Sublingual immunotherapy in asthma and rhinoconjunctivitis: systematic review of paediatric literature. Arch Dis Child [article on the Internet] 2004 [cited January 2024], 89:620-4. Available from: https://adc.bmj.com/content/89/7/620
51.-Olaguibel JM, Alvarez Puebla MJ. Efficacy of sublingual allergy vaccination for respiratory allergy in children. Conclusions from one meta-analysis. J Investig Allergol Clin Immunol [article on the Internet] 2005 [cited January 2024], 15:9-16. Available from: https://pubmed.ncbi.nlm.nih.gov/15864877/
Penagos M, Compalati E, Tarantini F, Passalacqua G, Canonica GW. Efficacy of sublingual immunotherapy in the treatment of allergic rhinitis in pediatric patients 3 to 18 years of age: a meta-analysis of randomized, placebo- controlled, double-blind trials. Ann Allergy Asthma Immunol [article on the Internet].

2006 [cited January 2024], 97:141-8. Available from: https://pubmed.ncbi.nlm.nih.gov/16937742/
Penagos M, Passalacqua G, Compalati E, Baena-Cagnani CE, Orozco S, Pedroza A, et al. Meta-analysis of the efficacy of sublingual immunotherapy in the treatment of allergic asthma in pediatric patients, 3 to 18 years of age. Chest [article on the Internet] 2008 [cited January 2024], 133:599-609. Available from: https://pubmed.ncbi.nlm.nih.gov/17951626/
54.-Roder E, Berger MY, de Groot H, van Wiik RG. Immunotherapy in

children and adolescents with allergic rhinoconjunctivitis: a systematic review. Pediatr Allergy Immunol [article on the Internet] 2008 [cited Jan. 2024], 19:197-
207. Available at: https://www.ncbi.nlm.nih.gov/books/NBK75661/

55.-Corrigan CJ, Kettner J, Doemer C, Cromwell O. Efficacy and safety of pre-seasonal specific immunotherapy with a six-herb pollen allergoid adsorbed on aluminium. Allergy. [article on the Internet] 2005 [cited on January from 2024]; The 60:801-807. Available en:
http://www.scielo.org.mx/scielo.php?script=sci_arttext&pid=S2448-
91902020000400309
56.-Lichtenstein LM, Marismeño DG. Efficacy and safety of long-term ragweed allergoid treatment. J Allergy Clin Immunol [article on the Internet] 1981 [cited January 2024]; 68:460-470. Available from:
https://karger.com/kxn/article/4/2/58/824926/Inmunoterapia-con-
alergenos-
para-diseases

57.-Potter PC. Update 0n sublingual Immunotherapy; Ann Allergy Clin Immunol [article on the Internet] 2006 [cited January 2024]; 96, No. 2; Suppl 1: S22. Available from: https://pubmed.ncbi.nlm.nih.gov/16496508/
Niederberger V, Horak F, Vrtala S, Spitzauer S, Krauth Montana, et al. Vaccination with genetically engineered allergens prevents progression of allergic disease. Proc Natl Acad Sci USA. [article on the Internet] 2004 [cited at January from 2024]; The 101:14677-14682. Available at:
https://www.elsevier.es/es-revista-allergologia-et-immunopathologia-105-
articulo-genetics-allergy-13003901
59.-Gefter Massachusett, et al. Treatment of cat allergy with T-cell reactive peptides. J Respir Crit Care Med. [article on the Internet] 1996 [cited January 2024];154:1623-1628.Available from:

https://karger.com/kxn/article/4/2/58/824926/Inmunoterapia-con-
alergenos- para-diseases
Marcucci F, Sensi L, Frati F, Senna GE, Canonica, GW, Parmiani S, Passalacqua G. Sublingual tryptase and DBS in children treated with grass pollen sublingual immunotherapy (SLIT): safety and immunologic implications. Allergy [article on the Internet] 2001 [cited January 2024]; 56: 1091-5. Available from: https://pubmed.ncbi.nlm.nih.gov/11703225/
Drachenberg KJ, Wheeler AW, Stuebner P, Horak F. Allergy. [article on the Internet] 2001 [cited January 2024]; 56:498-505. Available from:

https://pubmed.ncbi.nlm.nih.gov/11421893/
62.-Schroeder JT, Hamilton RG, Balcer-Whaley SL, Khattignavong AP, et al. Immunotherapy with a Toll-like ragweed receptor 9 agonist vaccine for allergic rhinitis. N Engl J Med. [article on the Internet] 2006 [cited Jan 2024]; The 355:1445-1455. Available at: https://www.nejm.org/doi/full/10.1056/NEJMoa052916
63.-Malling H, Weeke B. Immunotherapy Position paper of the European Academy of Allergology and Clinicals Immunology. Allergy [article on the Internet] 1993 [cited on January 2024]; 48, suppl 14. Available from: https://hub.eaaci.org/resources/position-papers/
64.-Malling H-J. Immunotherapy as an effective tool in allergy treatment. Allergy [article on the Internet] 2008 [cited January 2024]; 53:461-472. Available at:https://acaai.org/allergies/management-treatment/allergy-immunotherapy/#:~:text=Overview,which%20the%20person%20is%20allergic. 65.-Bousquet J,Lockey RF, Malling H-J. WHO Position Paper: Allergenimmunotherapy: Therapeutic vaccines for allergic diseases. Allergy [article on the Internet] 1998 [cited January 2024]; 53:1-49. Available from: https://www.jacionline.org/article/S0091-6749(98)70271-4/fulltext
66.-Ross RN, Nelson HS, Finegold I. Effectiveness of specific immunotherapyin the treatment of asthma: a meta-analysis of prospective, randomized, double-blind, placebo-controlled studies. ClinTher [article in Internet] 2000; 22:329-341. Available at: https://pubmed.ncbi.nlm.nih.gov/10963287/

Lorente Toledano F, Laffond E, Moreno E, Dávila I. Therapeutic Vaccines in Respiratory Allergy: Are they effective? La Alergia Clin Exp. [article on the Internet] 2006 [cited on January 2024]; El 22:34-54. Available from:

https://www.cun.es/enfermedades-tratamientos/tratamientos/inmunoterapia- allergology
68.-Pérez Martín J. Immunotherapy subcutaneous allergen-specific immunotherapy in patients with asthma and allergic rhinitis. Siglo XXI. Revista Alergia México [article on the Internet] 2009 [cited January 2024]; 56(2):27-29. Available from: http://www.scielo.org.mx/scielo.php?script=sci_arttext&pid=S2448-91902019000300301
Martínez Jiménez NE, Aguilar Ángeles D., Rojas Ramos E. Prevalence

of sensitization to Blomia tropicalis and Dermatophagoides pteronyssinus, farinae and siboney in patients with rhinitis or allergic asthma (or both) in a population of the metropolitan area of Mexico City. Revista Alergia México [article on the Internet] 2010 [cited January 2024]; 57(1):3-10. Available from: https://www.imbiomed.com.mx/articulo.php?id=62119

70.- Ferrer Alemán E. Subcutaneous immunotherapy with mites in allergic patients. [Thesis] Work to opt for the title of first degree specialist in Allergology. Santiago de Cuba: Higher Institute of Medical Sciences; 2011.

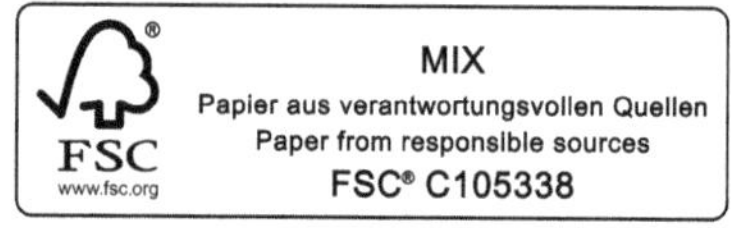

Printed by Books on Demand GmbH, Norderstedt / Germany